FAST Liver Cleanse and Detox Diet

Remove Toxins, Cleanse Your Liver, and Improve Your Health

By Lucas Strong

Published in Canada

© Copyright 2015 – Lucas Strong

ISBN-13: 978-1508669197
ISBN-10: 1508669198

Table of Contents

Introduction 1

Chapter 1: The Importance of Cleansing and Detoxing 3

    The Difference Between a Cleanse and a Detox ..4

    How a Detox Diet Works 5

    The Importance of a Liver Cleanse.........................7

Chapter 2: Understanding the Liver Cleansing Process 9

    Getting to Know Your Liver 9

    How a Liver Cleanse Works...................................10

    The Benefits of the Liver Cleanse.........................12

    Super Foods for the Liver 12

    "Anti-Liver" Foods to Avoid.................................13

Chapter 3: The Side Effects to Expect 15

Chapter 4: The Standard Liver Cleanse and Detox Diet 17

    Shop for the Super Foods 17

    Start with a Colon and Kidney Cleanse 18

    Variations of the Liver Cleanse.............................18

    Move on to a Liver Detox Tea 21

Chapter 5: Liver Cleanse and Detox Shortcuts.......23

    Liver Cleanse Shortcut...23

    Liver Cleanse and Detox Shortcut 24

Conclusion..27

Introduction

Our bodies are deteriorating at a much faster rate due to the increasing amount of toxins in our environment. While we have the science and technology to alleviate the symptoms caused by the poisons that enter our organs daily, but these medicines and treatments are merely temporary. If we continue going about our lives consuming unhealthy foods, alcohol, or drugs, the symptoms will remain. Moreover, drugs taken regularly to alleviate the pain also pose a threat to our system.

Our liver is the first defense against toxins that enter our bodies. However, because we continuously dump toxins into our bodies, the liver will deteriorate and eventually fail. So, what can be done to help the liver?

The answer starts with a liver cleanse and detox diet. This is an essential step towards recharging the liver and eliminating any traces of toxins within it. Thereafter it is important to make an effort to live a healthy lifestyle.

This book will help you give your liver a brand new start by including an overview of a cleanse and detox program, and specific steps on how carry it out. It is important to note that individuals with medical issues such as diabetes or an existing liver problem should consult their doctor before undergoing any sort of at-home treatment. You have no better time than now to save your liver from cancer before it's too late.

Chapter 1:
The Importance of Cleansing and Detoxing

Our world is becoming more toxic with each passing day. Everything, from the food we eat, to the water we drink and bathe in, to the air that we breathe, is contaminated with toxins from chemical factories. For example, a study of placenta from newborn babies showed traces of lead, mercury, and other toxic substances. We are born into it. Toxins cause most, if not all, of the illnesses we suffer from, including allergies and cancer.

If we make a conscious effort to regularly cleanse and detoxify our bodies, we can greatly reduce the risk of disease. Moreover this habit can make you look and feel healthy and happy. In fact, a regular cleanse and detox has become so effective that it has become a big trend, particularly in the entertainment industry where health and beauty are the focus. For instance, Beyonce Knowles lauded the detox diet for helping her get rid of 20 pounds, over 9 kilograms, when she was filming the movie "Dreamgirls."

For those performing a cleanse or detox for the first time, it is important to fully understand the benefits as well as the risks that come with them. Keep in mind that celebrities are guided by a medical and fitness professional while they are carrying out their cleanse and detox.

The Difference Between a Cleanse and a Detox

The terms "cleanse" and "detox" may cause confusion, especially since they often used synonymously. The main reason for this is that most of the methods in a *detox* plan can also be found in a *cleanse* plan. For the sake of clarity, there is a fine line between the two, with the main difference in the results you want to obtain.

Detoxing has been practiced for hundreds of years in different countries across the world. When you detox the body, you make a decision to undergo a certain procedure or diet to purge the toxins from your system. Detox is short for "detoxification," and it is defined as a treatment for poison carried out by neutralizing the toxic properties. It typically involves the normal functioning of the liver. You eliminate many common foods from your diet, including soft drinks and fast food. Any foods containing even a small amount of toxins should be avoided, or all your efforts will be in vain.

Conversely, when you cleanse the body, while you are also undergoing a diet restriction, here it is for the sake of eliminating waste from the body, especially from the digestive system. During a cleanse, lifestyle changes are not as drastic as compared to a detox. For instance, a liver cleanse only requires one to drink a hot cup of dandelion root tea before going to bed.

How a Detox Diet Works

Generally speaking, a will person detox when he or she needs to overcome a particular addiction, such as drugs or alcohol abuse, smoking, or overconsumption of food. The poisons a detox seeks to neutralize include more than the kinds found under one's kitchen sink. Several products we use or consume contain levels of "poisons" that are deemed "safe" because the amounts are too insignificant to cause harm to the body. Nevertheless, if we constantly consume these products, we build up the amount of poisons in our body which are difficult, at times impossible, to eliminate without the help of a detox diet. A detox diet is highly restrictive. You have to avoid many foods and beverages that are known for containing toxins. Because of this restrictive nature, medical professionals only allow their patients to undergo a detox diet plan for a limited amount of time. Furthermore, it is mandatory for individuals who have medical issues to consult a doctor prior to engaging in any sort of dietary plan.

The most common detox diet is implemented over 13 days. The first three days consists of an all-liquid fast limited to water, lemon water, or tea. On the fourth day, the dieter transitions to a 10-day vegetable and fruit diet with highly controlled portions.Following the 13 day detox diet plan, the dieter will then move on to a paleolithic diet, consisting of eating strictly whole, raw food.

A person serious about ridding his or her body of toxins should avoid tobacco, drugs, caffeine, and alcohol, along with processed foods and supplements. He or she should stick to eating organic fruits and vegetables and whole or raw nuts and grains since these foods are guaranteed to be free from pesticides and other poisons. Certain foods such as purified water, herbs and lemon juice help aid in the overall detox plan. A major risk posed by a detox diet, however, is its substantial lack of protein.When you undergo a detox diet plan, you are also advised to follow an overall body cleansing plan. To meet this element, some dieters will sauna or sometimes even take laxatives or receive enemas to help boost the effectiveness of their plan.

The Importance of a Liver Cleanse

While a detox mainly concerns eliminating toxins from the whole body, a cleanse can be more focused on a specific part of the body you want to treat. The main focus from here on will be liver cleansing.The liver acts as your body's first line of defense against toxins by filtering them out and preventing their entry into the blood stream. There is a great deal of information you need to learn and understand about how a liver cleanse works The next chapter will discuss the importance of a liver cleanse for your health.

Chapter 2:
Understanding the Liver
Cleansing Process

There are several options to choose from when it comes to cleansing and detoxification programs. However, if you have to choose one, then you might want to consider the liver cleanse.

Getting to Know Your Liver

The liver weighs approximately 49 ounces (or 1.4 kilograms) and is around 8 to 9 inches (or 20 to 23 centimeters) in diameter. It is one of the most vital, and likely the most abused, internal organ. People do not usually think or even care about the liver until it starts to malfunction. Failure to care for your liver will result in serious degenerative illnesses which are usually irreversible.

The liver is your body's natural detoxification system. It has the ability to break down toxins and prevent them from entering your blood stream, to produce bile for better food digestion, to store energy in the form of glucose, and to metabolize fats and proteins.

When the liver is overloaded with overly processed foods that contain high amounts of toxins, preservatives, pesticides, and additives, it starts to malfunction. Symptoms of a damaged liver include high cholesterol and triglyceride levels, malnutrition, gallstones, and allergies.

How a Liver Cleanse Works

There are different methods for performing a liver cleanse, and the main differences are usually based in the length of time given for each stage during the process. However, the general details stay the same.

The first stage of the liver cleanse involves fasting. This process eliminates any traces of toxins that are still inside your system, particularly your liver. The only intake allowed includes water and herbal teas. The fast usually lasts for 48 hours. For some variations, the faster can drink fresh juices such as apple or lemon juice along with specific amounts of olive oil and Epsom salts.

Stage two involves a gradual transition back to solid foods by eating raw fruits and vegetables. The dieter should allow himself or herself a span of 7 to 10 days before re-introducing cooked foods. This re-introduction should also be done gradually, starting with one cooked meal for every 24 hours. Most variations of the cleanse recommends the individual maintain the habit of regularly drinking herbal tea, especially dandelion root and milk thistle.

Keep in mind that you might experience feelings of nausea and sometimes even vomiting while in the middle of your liver cleanse because of the drastic change in your diet and the purging of toxins from your body. Additionally, women who are about to, or are in the middle of, their monthly period should avoid doing the liver cleanse. The liver is doing nearly twice as much work during this time to help eliminate excess fluids from the body. Therefore, liver cleanse would only stress out the already busy organ. Finally most people who choose to do a liver cleanse also undergo a colon cleanse because most experts say that one cannot be fully effective without the other.

Individuals who are uncomfortable with a highly restrictive diet usually resort to alternatives to liver cleansing, such as acupuncture or the use of essential oils on the skin or in hot tea.

The Benefits of the Liver Cleanse

The most obvious benefit of a liver cleanse would be a toxin-free liver. It is almost like resetting your body back to when you were a healthy, young child. A healthier liver means a healthier immune system as well. You will notice that any previous ailments that you have had in the past are gone, such as gall stones, allergies, and hepatitis. The liver cleanse will also regulate your blood sugar and body fat and boost amino acids. Apart from an improved overall wellbeing, the liver cleanse can also alleviate body pain, nausea and fatigue. You will feel more energized and happy. Lastly, people who complete the entire liver cleansing process will be able to form healthy habits and be rid of certain addictions, ultimately making them healthier and more disciplined.

Super Foods for the Liver

Nature has provided certain foods that can help improve and maintain the health of your liver. You can juice these foods during the initial stages of your cleanse, and eat them raw or steamed once you have started introducing solid foods back into your diet. These super foods for your liver include broccoli, artichokes, cauliflower, beets, carrots, cabbage, wild greens, and sprouts. These foods have high amounts of fiber, zinc, and vitamins C and E.

"Anti-Liver" Foods to Avoid

Foods that have been overly processed contain too many chemicals, additives and preservatives, making them even more difficult for the liver to process. Some examples include sugary foods and foods that are too high in fat and sodium. Furthermore, you should greatly limit your intake of caffeine and alcohol, or better yet avoid them altogether. It is important to know that alcohol is one of the main causes of liver failure.

Chapter 3:
The Side Effects to Expect

With a solid understanding of how a liver cleanse and detox diet works, one can start preparing a program that he or she wishes to follow. Remember that it is highly recommended to consult a medical professional prior to engaging in any sort of drastic procedures because such programs can be dangerous if not implemented correctly.

Before engaging in any sort of cleanse or detox, keep in mind the side effects that you will experience. Our body has become used to its somewhat toxic state such that it will at first react negatively to the cleanse. Certain parts of your body may exhibit strange and often uncomfortable symptoms because of the circulation of toxins that the system is gradually purging. For instance, if the toxins are being expelled through the pores of our skin, rashes are likely. Discoloration may also occur, although this is temporary. Additionally you might also emit a strange body odor because of the specific foods and liquids that you are consuming for cleansing and detoxification. Long term cleanse and detox programs can also trigger nausea and fatigue. Cleanse and detox diets that last longer, should cause significant weight loss. Another common side effect that most people experience during a cleanse and detox diet is insomnia.

This might be due to the chemical changes and readjustment of hormonal levels that the internal system is experiencing. The liquid-only stage of the detox diet will definitely trigger mood swings, so be prepared to have a will of iron during that time. Due to these possible side effects, it is highly advised that you schedule any type of cleanse and detox diet when you are not busy or about to do any sort of intensive activity.

Chapter 4:
The Standard Liver Cleanse and Detox Diet

This chapter is dedicated to showing you the entire process of a standard at-home liver cleanse and detox diet.

Shop for the Super Foods

In order to carry out a liver cleanse and detox, you will need lemons or lemon juice, garlic cloves, ginger root, flaxseed oil (cold pressed), cayenne pepper, acidophilus, Epsom salts, extra-virgin olive oil, ornithine capsules, milk thistle and dandelion root in tea or 120 mg capsule form, and cola. All of these items must be fresh and organic. Therefore it is important to carefully read the label and avoid any fruit cocktail varieties. . Try any reputable nutrition center or health food store in your area to purchase these items. Do plenty of research before buying anything online.

Start with a Colon and Kidney Cleanse

Once you have acquired all of the items you need for the diet, you must first undergo the cleanse before moving on to the detox diet. Most experts prescribe a colon cleanse as well as a kidney cleanse before the liver cleanse. If you wish to carry out a colon cleanse, consult a medical professional or do additional research. Finally, the liver cleanse is the most potent of the three so it is advised that your kidneys and colon are completely cleared out in order to minimize the stress inside your body.

Variations of the Liver Cleanse

There are two types of liver cleanses to choose from. To perform the first variation follow the seven steps below:

Step 1: Prepare lemon juice, with either three lemons or six tablespoons (90 ml) of lemon juice.

Step 2: Grate two garlic cloves and approximately two inches (5 cm) of fresh ginger root, and mix these thoroughly into your juice concoction. Garlic has highly potent, detoxifying, and anti-bacterial properties, while ginger boosts blood circulation.

Step 3: Add two tablespoons (30 ml) of cold pressed flaxseed oil. This oil contains Omega 3 fatty acids that will stabilize your liver's bile production.

Step 4: Add one teaspoon (5 ml) of acidophilus. This is an essential ingredient in the liver cleanse because it contains good bacteria that will stop your liver triglyceride levels from rising.

Step 5: Add a dash of cayenne pepper to stimulate your liver in purging the toxins out.

Step 6: Blend everything together into a smoothie. Drink this smoothie at 2:00 p.m., 6:00 p.m. and 8:00 p.m. Instead of repeating these steps three times a day, triple the amount in the recipe to create three servings within a single blend.

Step 7: Throughout the cleanse, eat one serving of fresh fruit during breakfast and lunch. Do not eat anything after 2 p.m. Expect more frequent trips to the bathroom during these times because the cleanse also acts as a laxative.

To perform the second variation of the liver cleanse, follow these steps:

Step 1: Squeeze the juice out of three to four large lemons or pour in six to nine tablespoons (90 to 105 ml) of lemon juice into a container.

Step 2: Add four tablespoons (60 ml) of magnesium sulfate or Epsom salts into the lemon juice and mix thoroughly. Epsom salts are a potent laxative that speed up the purging of toxins from the body.

Step 3: Pour in a one-half cup (118 ml) of extra-virgin olive oil. This will trigger bile production in the the liver and gall bladder.

Step 4: If you desire, pour in a one-half cup of cola. This makes drinking the mixture it easier.

Step 5: Blend the ingredients well before drinking the mixture. Also, make sure to drink it on an empty stomach. Eat one serving of fresh fruit during breakfast and lunch. You can have one additional serving of fresh fruit at 3:00 p.m. Drink the liver cleanse mixture exactly 4 hours after your last meal to ensure your stomach is empty.

Step 6: You may also take four orthinine capsules together while drinking this mixture. orthinine is a non-protein amino acid that aids with sleep so that you will not experience nausea after drinking the mixture.

Either one of these cleanses should be carried out during the weekend, preferably a Saturday, so that there is time to recover on Sunday.

Move on to a Liver Detox Tea

At the end of the liver cleanse, you must transition to a healthier lifestyle in order to maintain the effects of the purge. Start with a liquid diet of strictly purified water and liver detox tea for the first twelve to twenty-four hours after the cleanse.

To prepare the liver detox tea, you will need hepatic herbs, which specifically help improve the overall health of the liver. Hepatic herbs include dandelion root, prickly ash, milk thistle, yarrow, fennel, and yarrow. Other options are the mountain grape, hyssop, golden seal, wild indigo, horseradish, and motherwort herbs.

Keep in mind that the mountain grape, dandelion root and ash herbs also aid in the cleansing of your blood and boost your metabolism. You can find several tea blends specifically for liver detoxification in many health food stores. For safety reasons, make sure to do your research on the tea manufacturers beforehand.

To prepare the tea, you need boiling water. If the tea water is cold or room temperature, it will not work. Steep the tea leaves for three to five minutes or as based on the manufacturer's instructions before you sip it. You may also add a dash of cayenne pepper or a few drops of freshly squeezed lemon juice.

At the end of your liquid diet, you can gradually transition back to solid foods. Start out eating one serving of fresh fruit for breakfast, lunch and dinner for twenty-four to forty-eight hours. Next, introduce fresh vegetables for the following twenty-for to forty-eight hours. From there, move on to soft foods such as grilled or steamed, lean protein – fish or tofu – before returning to your regular diet. Most people prefer to stick to a vegetarian or Paleolithic diet following the liver cleanse for health reasons.

A liver cleanse should only be performed once every twelve months due to its highly potent effects. If you feel that you need to carry out a second cleanse before the end of the twelve month period, you should consult a medical professional for guidance.

Chapter 5:
Liver Cleanse and Detox
Shortcuts

For those of you who cannot afford a regular liver cleanse and detox diet at the time, then this chapter is dedicated to you. While these are shorter variations of the liver cleanse, you can still enjoy the same benefits of the process so long as you transition to the detox diet afterward.

Liver Cleanse Shortcut

The shortcut liver cleanse involves apple juice and takes three das to complete. Additionally, all you will need is pure organic apple juice.On the first day, drink two glasses of apple juice every two hours, for a period of twelve hours. Do not eat or drink anything else except purified water.On the second day, continue to drink two glasses of apple juice every two hours, and then right before going to bed, drink a one-half cup of apple juice with one-half cup of extra-virgin olive oil.On the third and final day, squeeze out the juice from one lemon into one liter of water. Drink this lemon water gradually over a span of two to three hours. Following this three day cleanse, you can return to solid foods, preferably organic fruits and vegetables.

Liver Cleanse and Detox Shortcut

As you may have already noticed, detox diets take longer than cleanses. If you wish to carry out a shorter version of the diet, follow the instructions below. Keep in mind this diet will not be as potent as the standard version.

Additionally, seven days before performing the actual detox, you must limit your foods to: vegetables such as cabbage, broccoli, brussell sprouts, cauliflower, parsley, mustard greens, kale, dandelion greens, watercress, escarole, chard, beets, cilantro, artichokes, celery, and asparagus;fruits such as oranges, limes, lemons, apples, berries, carrots and pear; and foods rich in sulfur, such as onions, garlic, daikon radish and eggs.For your protein intake, eat two servings of lean chicken, turkey, fish, or beef. Vegetarians or vegans can opt for at least two tablespoons daily of premium quality spirulina or blue-green algae as an alternative.Along with these food options, take one to two tablespoons of olive or flaxseed oil. You should also consume one serving of powdered psyllium husks or ground flaxseeds with each meal.As for liquid intake, limit yourself to herbal tea and purified or filtered water. To determine the daily amount of water that you need to drink, measure your body weight in pounds and divide that number into two. Drink the amount that you get, in ounces.Avoid at all costs artificial sweeteners, gluten (from wheat, rye, barley, etc), refined carbohydrates (white flour, white rice, etc), alcohol, drugs and caffeine.After seven days, fast for one day limiting yourself to water and herbal tea. that the following week, mix cranberry water, fresh orange and lemon juice, cinnamon, nutmeg, ground ginger, and stevia herb.

After completing the seven-day restrictive diet and the day-long fast and juice drink, follow the steps below to complete the detox diet:

Step 1: Bring the cranberry water to a boil and then lower the heat.

Step 2: Add the nutmeg, cinnamon and ginger into the cranberry water and let simmer for fifteen to twenty minutes. Set aside until it is cooled to room temperature.

Step 3: Add orange and lemon juice along with stevia to the mixture.

Alternate drinking one cup (8 ounces) of filtered or purified water and one cup of the juice at least every sixty minutes throughout the day. You must drink at least 72 ounces of water and another 72 ounces of the juice.Make sure to take one to two teaspoons of powdered psyllium husks or two to three tablespoons of ground or milled flaxseeds, once in the morning and once at night, along with the water or juice.

After completing the 24-hour liver detox, limit your foods to the following over the subsequent three days: the foods were enumerated above in the 7-day pre-detox diet, and add nonfat yogurt. Also take 500 to 540 mgs of betaine hydrochloride, or 100 to 150 mgs of pepsin, along with 50 mgs of ox bile extract before each meal.

Conclusion

The liver cleanse and detox diet will produce outstanding effects for your health. However, the journey to a better, healthier life does not end with this program. Strive to take better care of your body each and every day. There will be times when you succumb to eating unhealthy foods containing toxins, but do not allow yourself to return to the dangerous and toxic path again. Every single day, you have the opportunity to live a healthy life. Keep track of your progress and constantly motivate yourself to stick to a clean routine.

Thank you for choosing this book, I hope it gave you a clear understanding of this topic and how to start your journey to a better, healthier you.

DISCLAIMER AND/OR LEGAL NOTICES: Every effort has been made to accurately represent this book and it's potential. Results vary with every individual, and your results may or may not be different from those depicted. No promises, guarantees or warranties, whether stated or implied, have been made that you will produce any specific result from this book. Your efforts are individual and unique, and may vary from those shown. Your success depends on your efforts, background and motivation.

The material in this publication is provided for educational and informational purposes only and is not intended as medical advice. The information contained in this book should not be used to diagnose or treat any illness, metabolic disorder, disease or health problem. Always consult your physician or health care provider before beginning any nutrition or exercise program. Use of the programs, advice, and information contained in this book is at the sole choice and risk of the reader.